RENAISSANCE FITNESS:

Unleashing Your Potential in the Modern Age

Anthony R. Lowry

TABLE OF CONTENTS

INTRODUCTION

CHAPTER 1: RENAISSANCE FITNESS

1.1 Defining a holistic approach to health:

1.2 Embracing a renaissance mindset:

CHAPTER 2: MINDFUL MOVEMENT PRACTICES

2.1 Exploring diverse forms of exercise:

2.2 The synergy between body and mind in movement:

CHAPTER 3: NUTRITION FOR OPTIMAL PERFORMANCE

3.1 Balancing traditional and contemporary dietary principles:

3.2 Superfoods and their impact on vitality:

CHAPTER 4: INTEGRATING ANCIENT PRACTICES

4.1 Yoga, tai chi, and other timeless disciplines:

4.2 Adapting ancient wisdom to modern lifestyles:

CHAPTER 5: TECH-ASSISTED WELLNESS

5.1 Wearables and smart devices for fitness tracking:

5.2 Apps and tools for personalized wellness plans:

CHAPTER 6: MIND-BODY CONNECTION

6.1 The role of mental well-being in physical fitness:

6.2 Mindfulness and stress management for overall health:

CHAPTER 7: FUNCTIONAL FITNESS FOR EVERYDAY LIFE

7.1 Building strength and mobility for real-world scenarios:

7.2 Practical exercises for functional fitness:

CHAPTER 8: SLEEP SCIENCE AND RECOVERY

8.1 Optimizing sleep for physical and mental recovery:

8.2 The impact of sleep on overall well-being:

CHAPTER 9: BIOHACKING FOR PEAK PERFORMANCE

9.1 Nootropics, supplements, and biohacking techniques:

9.2 Responsible and ethical biohacking practices:

CHAPTER 10: CREATING YOUR RENAISSANCE FITNESS LIFESTYLE

10.1 Developing a personalized fitness and wellness routine:

10.2 Sustaining long-term health and vitality:

CONCLUSION

INTRODUCTION

Welcome to a transforming journey in which the echoes of ancient wisdom blend with the rhythms of modern life. The search for health and vitality has taken center stage in the frantic symphony of our fast-paced world. This book, "Renaissance Fitness: Unleashing Your Potential in the Modern Age," challenges you to become the architect of your own well-being, combining timeless concepts from the past with cutting-edge technologies from the present.

We are on the cusp of a rebirth in the realization that fitness is something that people should pursue outside of the gym. Drawing from the diverse wisdom of ancient cultures, this renaissance celebrates the symbiosis between body and mind.

The adventure we start on is a comprehensive quest for healthy living, not just an investigation of workout regimens or food programs. "Renaissance Fitness" is a book that will help you negotiate the complexity of modern life while honoring the underlying pillars of well-being that have lasted the test of time.

In the next chapters, we will unravel the fabric of Renaissance Fitness, investigating varied movement methods that reflect the elegance of ancient disciplines and uncovering dietary concepts that feed not only physical power but long-term vitality. We'll look at the intersection of technology and wellness, as well as the power of mindful movement and the fundamental link between mental and physical health.

This is more than a book; it's an invitation.

CHAPTER 1: RENAISSANCE FITNESS

Renaissance Fitness is a revolutionary journey that will unlock the entire range of your physical and mental talents. In an era marked by development and invention, our approach to exercise goes beyond the norm, representing the spirit of the Renaissance - a resurgence of strength, energy, and a harmonic balance of mind and body.

Our philosophy at Renaissance Fitness is to shape not only bodies but also destinies. In this modern age, where demands on our time and energy are relentless, we serve as architects of a healthier, more resilient you. We guarantee that you will not only reach but surpass your fitness objectives with our philosophy, which is a celebration of the human spirit and a blend of traditional knowledge and modern science.

Step inside our sanctuary, where the air is imbued with a sense of growth, and the decor vibrates with inspiration.

Our cutting-edge facilities are intended to meet every facet of your fitness journey, creating an environment that fosters growth, persistence, and self-discovery. We are dedicated to pushing the boundaries of what you believe is possible, from beautifully designed exercise environments to new training approaches.

On this transforming journey, our team of committed and motivated fitness specialists will act as your mentors. We use a holistic approach, drawing inspiration from the Renaissance, and recognize that genuine fitness includes not just physical fitness but also mental and emotional well-being. Personalized exercise regimens, dietary advice, and mindfulness techniques all come together to equip you to embrace a modern-day lifestyle.

At Renaissance Fitness, we comprehend that your true capacity is endless. We think of fitness as an art form, a surface on which you can create a masterpiece out of your own strength, resilience, and vitality. Our responsibility is to give you the apparatuses, information, and backing expected to explore the difficulties of the cutting-edge age with force and beauty.

Join us as we set out on this journey, and allow Renaissance Fitness to serve as the impetus for your own recuperation. Discover your latent potential, escape the confines of the norm, and create a future that is bright, strong, and entirely your own. Renaissance Fitness believes that your potential is unlimited, so come change the story of your own physical and mental prowess in this era of limitless possibilities.

1.1 Defining a holistic approach to health:

A holistic approach to health emerges as a bright tapestry in the kaleidoscope of human well-being, carefully woven with strands of physical vigor, mental clarity, emotional harmony, and spiritual resonance. It is a sophisticated philosophy that surpasses reductionist thinking by embracing the full individual in all of their features and dimensions. The holistic approach directs a harmonic melody in the big symphony of life, directing a dance of interrelated components that together build the exquisite composition of genuine health.

The holistic approach to health, at its core, sees the individual as a dynamic and interconnected whole, with the flourishing of one part resonating across the entire system. It represents a shift away from the fragmented viewpoints that separate body from mind, emotion from physiology, and recognizes that the human experience is a complex tapestry of linked aspects, each affecting and shaping the others.

The holistic lens reveals a perspective of the body as a precious vessel deserving of sustenance, exercise, and care in the world of physical well-being. Nutrition has evolved beyond simply subsistence to become a tool for empowerment and healing. Holistic health values the body as a living, breathing creature worthy of thoughtful care and a healthy interaction with its surroundings, rather than as a machine.

Under the umbrella of holistic health, mental and emotional well-being becomes a delicate dance of self-discovery and acceptance. Mindfulness evolves from a catchphrase to a way of being, a practice that peels back the layers of the mind to bring one into the present moment. Emotional intelligence takes center stage, supporting the genuine expression and comprehension of one's emotions while also building resilience and inner balance.

In the social domain, holistic health exposes the enormous influence of interpersonal connections on an individual's well-being. Relationships become more than simply a way of life; they become a cornerstone of health, providing support, companionship, and a sense of belonging. In its different manifestations, the community becomes a caring environment in which the seeds of happiness can take root and develop.

As the holistic approach recognizes the delicate dance between human health and the well-being of the earth, environmental issues take on new relevance. A sustainable and healthy environment becomes a personal responsibility, acknowledging that the air we breathe, the water we drink, and the spaces we live in are all important to our total health.

In the spiritual and existential dimensions, the holistic approach invites individuals to explore the depths of their inner selves. It encourages the alignment of actions with personal values, fostering a sense of purpose that transcends the mundane. Connection to something greater, whether it be a spiritual belief, a sense of wonder, or an existential understanding, becomes a wellspring of resilience and inspiration.

Preventive healthcare, within the holistic paradigm, transforms into a proactive and empowered stance. Regular check-ups and screenings become not just precautionary measures but affirmations of self-care, acknowledging that health is not merely the absence of illness but a dynamic state of balance and vitality.

Lifelong learning, as an integral component of holistic health, becomes a perpetual journey of intellectual stimulation and personal growth. The mind, like the body, craves nourishment, and the pursuit of knowledge becomes a source of mental resilience and a pathway to a richer, more fulfilling life.

Finally, the holistic approach to health is a celebration of life's delicate dance, recognizing that genuine well-being includes the physical, mental, emotional, social, environmental, and spiritual elements. It is an invitation to engage on a journey of self-discovery, empowerment, and connection—to embrace the symphony of their own existence and delight in the pleasant melodies of holistic health.

1.2 Embracing a renaissance mindset:

Adopting a Renaissance mindset is analogous to opening the shutters of your consciousness to the great array of possibilities that life has to offer. It's an encouragement to create a diverse attitude to life, gaining inspiration from the Renaissance's intellectual and cultural enthusiasm. Individuals who embrace this perspective traverse the current terrain with a feeling of curiosity, inventiveness, and a deep awareness of the interconnection of information.

1. Curiosity as a Catalyst:

Make curiosity your driving force in your pursuits. A Renaissance attitude fosters voracious curiosity—a yearning for knowledge that crosses disciplines. Consider each day to be a blank canvas waiting to be painted with the brushstrokes of adventure and discovery.

2. Interdisciplinary Thinking:

Break down the silos of conventional thinking. In the spirit of the Renaissance, cultivate an interdisciplinary approach to problem-solving and innovation. Recognize the inherent connections between seemingly disparate fields, allowing ideas to cross-pollinate and flourish in novel and unexpected ways.

3. Continuous Learning and Growth:

Adopt a lifetime learning commitment. Let each day be a chance for personal and intellectual progress, just as the Renaissance was an age of intellectual renewal. Seek out fresh information, engage in other points of view, and allow the search for wisdom to be a never-ending adventure.

4. Creative Expression as a Lifestyle:

Unleash your inner artist. Infuse creativity into all aspects of your life, whether via traditional arts, sciences, or everyday tasks. Approach problems with a creative mindset, seeking unique solutions that transcend the every day and inspire people around you.

5. Accepting Change and Adaptability:

Accept change as a necessary aspect of progress. Being flexible and resilient in the face of changing circumstances is part of a Renaissance attitude. Accept change as a chance for renewal, refinement, and the development of new possibilities, rather than as a source of disturbance.

6. Cultivating Critical Thinking:

Improve your analytical abilities. Critical thinking was essential throughout the Renaissance. Develop your capacity to question, evaluate, and decipher information. Approach difficulties with a critical eye, emphasizing intellectual rigor as a pillar of decision-making.

7. Balancing Tradition and Innovation:

Blend tradition with innovation. Just as the Renaissance artists revitalized classical themes with a contemporary twist, find the delicate balance between honoring traditions and fostering innovation. Merge the timeless with the avant-garde, creating a dynamic synthesis that propels you forward.

8. Global Perspective and Cultural Appreciation:

Embrace a global outlook. In the Renaissance, a broader understanding of the world fueled creativity. Appreciate and learn from diverse cultures, recognizing the richness that comes from a global perspective. Let cultural appreciation be a source of inspiration and unity.

9. Humanism and Compassionate Leadership:

Embody the humanist spirit. In a Renaissance mindset, compassion and empathy are not just virtues but guiding principles. Lead with a humane touch, valuing the well-being of individuals and communities. Let your actions reflect a commitment to the betterment of humanity.

10. Purposeful Living and Legacy Building:

Live with purpose and leave a legacy. Accept the notion that your activities contribute to a larger story. Strive to leave a good and enduring impression, whether via your career, relationships, or contributions to society—a legacy that recalls the Renaissance ethos of leaving the world a better place.

Living with a Renaissance mindset is essentially accepting that life is a work of art, a blank canvas that requires ongoing investigation, inventiveness, and intellectual vigor. The goal is to imbue every day with the spirit of the Renaissance, when the quest for knowledge, the appreciation of artistic expression, and the development of an integrated and interconnected worldview are not merely goals but rather the foundation of a happy and meaningful life.

CHAPTER 2: MINDFUL MOVEMENT PRACTICES

The notion of Renaissance Fitness arises as a beacon of enlightenment in the middle of the current age's hustle and bustle when the unrelenting pace of life often leaves us craving for moments of quiet and self-discovery. It goes beyond the traditional limitations of exercise, providing a comprehensive approach to physical well-being that extends beyond physical activity. Mindful Movement Practices, a transformational journey that invites individuals to embark on a voyage of self-discovery and unlock their latent potential, is at its core.

Renaissance Fitness challenges us to slow down, reconnect with our bodies, and embrace the practice of mindfulness in a society driven by quick cures and rapid satisfaction. It is a movement celebration that goes beyond the mechanical repetitions of traditional exercise and into the realms of self-awareness and conscious life. The core of this fitness revolution is molding the mind as well as the body, encouraging a harmonic marriage of physical and mental well-being.

Movement with Intention Renaissance Fitness practices is a symphony of intentional and purposeful movements that engage the body, mind, and soul. Each movement becomes a holy expression of self-discovery, whether it is via the elegant flow of yoga, the contemplative strides of Tai Chi, or the rhythmic dance of mindful aerobics. It's an invitation to discover the untapped reservoirs of strength, flexibility, and resilience that exist inside us and are just waiting to be discovered.

The ethos of Renaissance Fitness lies in embracing movement as a form of self-expression, a canvas upon which we paint the masterpiece of our own physical and mental well-being. In a society that often emphasizes the destination over the journey, this paradigm shift encourages us to revel in the present moment, finding joy in the rhythmic pulse of our heartbeat and the flowing breath that sustains us.

As we navigate the intricacies of our modern lives, Renaissance Fitness stands as a sanctuary, providing a refuge from the noise and chaos. It is a mindful oasis where individuals can reconnect with their inner selves, rediscover forgotten passions, and unfold the layers of their potential. In this renaissance, fitness becomes a sacred ritual, a daily affirmation of self-love and self-care.

Unleashing one's potential in the present day necessitates more than just physical power; it necessitates a harmonic combination of body, mind, and soul. Renaissance Fitness invites us to break free from the constraints of traditional workout regimens and embark on a transforming path of comprehensive well-being. Mindful Movement Practices not only shape our bodies but also pave the way for a more vivid and satisfying existence.

Every movement is a brushstroke in the Renaissance Fitness tapestry, every breath a note, and every attentive stride a dance of release. It is a hymn to the human spirit, a statement that our potential in the current day is not limited by cultural conventions or external expectations. Instead, it is a limitless energy waiting to be unleashed through the attentive and deliberate investigation of movement, in a renaissance that embraces the beauty of the human experience in all of its manifestations.

2.1 Exploring diverse forms of exercise:

It's like discovering a treasure trove of mental and physical health when you start exploring different types of exercise. Every distinct discipline offers a chance to not only improve our physical fitness but also to discover new limits within ourselves in a world where there is an abundance of movement modalities to choose from. Discovering the joy of movement in all its forms is invited by the diverse range of exercises, which includes the calm domains of yoga, the dynamic landscapes of martial arts, and the pulsating beats of dance.

Yoga, with its ancient wisdom origins, invites us to the mat for a complete examination of mind, body, and spirit. Yoga is a transforming practice that fosters flexibility, strength, and inner balance, whether practiced in the tranquil embrace of Hatha, the energetic sequences of Vinyasa, or the introspective journey of Yin. It is an internal journey in which each asana transforms into a meditation stance and the breath acts as a continuous companion on the path to self-discovery.

With their rich histories and various ideologies, martial arts enable practitioners to tap into their inner strength and create discipline, focus, and perseverance. Martial arts are a celebration of the body's potential for power and agility, from the flowing motions of Tai Chi, which resemble nature's dance, to the explosive kicks and punches of Muay Thai. The dojo, or training room, is transformed into a hallowed sanctuary for human development, where the martial artist learns not just to defend but also to embody the values of respect, humility, and persistence.

Dance, in all of its forms, provides a rhythmic celebration of self-expression and creativity. Dance surpasses the confines of traditional fitness, converting movement into an art form, from the elegance of ballet to the throbbing intensity of hip-hop. It is a channel through which people may connect with their emotions, let go of inhibitions, and relish in the simple thrill of moving to the beat. Dance is a vivid expression of the human spirit, not just an exercise.

CrossFit, a modern combination of many workout methods, tests the limits of strength, endurance, and adaptability. CrossFit aspires to create a well-rounded athlete capable of confronting any physical challenge through its high-intensity workouts and emphasis on functional movements. CrossFit's community element creates camaraderie and support, transforming fitness into a shared journey that transcends individual achievements.

Nature-based activities, such as hiking, trail running, or outdoor calisthenics, offer a refreshing escape from the confines of traditional gym settings. The great outdoors becomes a playground for physical exploration, where the uneven terrain and natural elements become the resistance for a full-body workout. Connecting with nature while engaging in physical activity adds an extra layer of invigoration to the exercise experience.

Pilates, with its emphasis on core strength, stability, and controlled movements, provides a low-impact yet highly effective approach to full-body conditioning. Pilates fosters an awareness of the body's alignment and encourages precise, flowing movements that enhance flexibility and build a strong foundation.

The joy of experimenting with different types of exercise is the breadth of experience and the ability to discover what best fits one's personal interests and goals. Whether you're looking for mindfulness in yoga, discipline in martial arts, creative expression in dance, or all-around fitness in CrossFit, each modality offers the door to a world of physical and mental well-being. The goal is to accept variation, listen to your body's messages, and see exercise as a lifetime experience.

2.2 The synergy between body and mind in movement:

The symbiotic relationship that exists between the mind and body when they move together is a fascinating dance of interdependence, in which the mental and physical realms come together to produce a cohesive whole. It is a deep partnership that goes beyond the simple performance of physical tasks, exploring the domains of awareness, mindfulness, and the complex conversation between the body and brain.

1. Embodied Cognition:

The central idea of the synergy is embodied cognition, which holds that the mind is not limited to the brain but rather permeates the entire body. Every thought materializes as a movement, and every movement is an embodiment of thought. In its graceful or dynamic expression, the body serves as a conduit for the mind's interaction with the outside world.

2. Mindful Movement:

When there is mindful movement, there is a strong sense of unity because each gesture and step is infused with conscious awareness. Whether it's the methodical flow of yoga, the accuracy of martial arts, or the graceful rhythm of dance, conscious movement transforms into a kind of meditation that strengthens the bond between the mental and physical domains.

3. Stress Reduction and Emotional Release:

Movement serves as a conduit for the release of pent-up emotions and stress. The mind, through the body's movement, can liberate itself from the burdens it carries. Whether it's the cathartic release of a sprint, the fluidity of dance, or the meditative pace of a walk, movement becomes a therapeutic journey that allows the mind to unwind and rejuvenate.

4. Neurotransmitters and Mood Enhancement:

Physical activity triggers the release of neurotransmitters such as endorphins, dopamine, and serotonin, influencing mood and cognitive function. The synergy between body and mind in movement becomes a natural mood enhancer, lifting spirits, reducing anxiety, and creating a sense of well-being.

5. Enhanced Cognitive Function:

The movement has been linked to improved cognitive function. The increased blood flow and oxygenation that accompany physical activity nourish the brain, enhancing concentration, memory, and overall cognitive abilities. The dynamic interplay between body and mind becomes a catalyst for mental acuity.

6. Flow State and Peak Performance:

The pinnacle of synergy is often experienced in the elusive state of flow, where movements become effortless, and the mind attains a heightened state of focus. Athletes, dancers, and artists alike tap into this harmonious collaboration, achieving peak performance as the boundaries between body and mind dissolve.

7. Posture and Confidence:

The connection between body and mind is reflected in posture and body language. As the body moves with strength and purpose, the mind follows suit, fostering confidence and a positive self-image. Conversely, mindful adjustments in posture can influence mental states, creating a feedback loop of empowerment.

8. Interoception and Body Awareness:

Interoception, the awareness of one's internal bodily sensations, is heightened through movement. The body becomes a canvas where the mind paints its sensations and feelings. This heightened body awareness nurtures a deeper understanding of oneself and promotes overall well-being.

9. Expressive Movement:

Movement serves as a language of expression, allowing the mind to communicate beyond the constraints of words. Whether in dance, sports, or other forms of physical activity, the body becomes a vessel for the articulation of emotions, thoughts, and the essence of the self.

10. Somatic Healing:

Physical and emotional traumas are addressed through movement as a means of somatic healing. Intentional, therapeutic movement can enhance the synergy between the body and mind, thereby promoting resilience and restoration and facilitating healing processes.

The synergy between the body and mind during movement is essentially an observance of the physical and mental domains' unbreakable union. It is an investigation of the deep conversation between the cognitive and the physical—a dance that goes beyond language barriers to open up a world of well-being, self-awareness, and the boundless possibilities of the human experience.

CHAPTER 3: NUTRITION FOR OPTIMAL PERFORMANCE

As the guiding light that illuminates the path toward optimal performance in the vibrant tapestry of our modern age, Renaissance Fitness stands out as a beacon of guidance. This life-changing experience is centered around the profound realization that optimal nutrition serves as the foundation for peak physical and mental performance.

In the labyrinth of contemporary challenges, the human body functions as a masterpiece, intricately designed and finely tuned. Just as a Renaissance artist meticulously crafts a timeless masterpiece, individuals seeking optimal performance must consider their bodies as the canvas awaiting the strokes of nutritional mastery. It is within this paradigm that Renaissance Fitness unfolds, inviting us to unleash our true potential through a symbiotic relationship with nutrition.

Fueling the body is not merely a routine but an art form, and the nutrients we ingest are the pigments that color our performance canvas. Nutritional science, akin to the palette of a master painter, offers a diverse array of elements, each playing a unique role in the symphony of optimal performance. Proteins, the structural architects; carbohydrates, the energy conductors; fats, the metabolic choreographers - together, they compose the harmonious composition of a finely tuned physique.

In the Renaissance Fitness narrative, micronutrients and antioxidants emerge as the unsung heroes, akin to the subtle brushstrokes that add depth and nuance to a masterpiece. Vitamins and minerals, like skilled artisans, fortify the body's intricate systems, ensuring that the symphony of performance resonates with vitality and resilience. Antioxidants, the guardians of cellular integrity, shield the body's citadel from the ravages of oxidative stress, allowing us to navigate the modern age with grace and vigor.

However, the Renaissance Fitness quest goes beyond the simple coordination of macronutrients and micronutrients. It invites us to build a conscious relationship with food, acknowledging the significant link between nutrition and mental health. As the Renaissance celebrated the beautiful blending of art and science, we must also recognize the subtle relationship between nutrition and cognitive performance.

Within Renaissance Fitness, staying hydrated is not just a routine chore but a ritual drink, an essential extract that keeps the body functioning. Similar to the inspiration sources that Renaissance intellectuals drew from, the elixir of water provides a steady supply of energy that keeps the wheels of performance turning.

The Renaissance Fitness concept challenges us to look beyond the commonplace ideas of diets and adopt a holistic view of nutrition as we set out to achieve peak performance. Instead of focusing on deprivation, the key is abundance: a surplus of flavors that delight, a surplus of nutrients that empower, and a surplus of vitality that embodies the full potential of humanity.

Renaissance Fitness provides a beacon of guidance in this day and age when striving for greatness is a joint effort by individuals and groups. It pushes us to reconsider how we relate to food, seeing it as a component of the work of art we are creating rather than as a means to an end. This work of art captures the symphony of our combined physical and mental abilities, the real embodiment of our freed potential in the contemporary era.

3.1 Balancing traditional and contemporary dietary principles:

Striking a delicate balance between the innovation of modern nutritional science and the wisdom of tradition is often necessary in the plethora of dietary options available in today's world in order to achieve optimal health. This balanced fusion of traditional and modern dietary practices is the cornerstone of a holistic approach to nutrition, acknowledging the enduring principles while adjusting to the changing demands of our active lives.

Traditional dietary wisdom, often rooted in cultural heritage and ancestral practices, lays the groundwork for understanding the intrinsic connection between food and well-being. Just as a seasoned gardener tends to the roots to ensure the vitality of the plant, traditional dietary principles emphasize the importance of whole, unprocessed foods - a timeless cornerstone that transcends generations. This includes an abundance of fruits, vegetables, whole grains, and lean proteins, embodying a holistic approach that mirrors the bountiful diversity found in nature.

In the rich tapestry of traditional diets, there exists a profound appreciation for locally sourced, seasonal ingredients – a practice that aligns with the innate rhythms of nature. This not only fosters a connection with the environment but also ensures a nutrient-rich, varied diet that adapts to the changing seasons, a principle that contemporary dietary approaches increasingly recognize and endorse.

On the other hand, modern times are advancing at an accelerated rate, bringing with them opportunities and challenges that call for a more sophisticated approach to eating. The role of particular nutrients, the intricacies of metabolism, and the customization of diets to meet individual needs are all clarified by modern nutritional science, which is comparable to a compass navigating unknown waters. As we explore the microbiome and uncover the mysteries of our genetic composition, a marriage of custom and innovation presents itself, providing individualized dietary plans that speak to the individuality of every person.

In the realm of contemporary dietary principles, there is a heightened awareness of dietary diversity not only in terms of whole foods but also in culinary techniques and global flavors. The fusion of traditional recipes with a modern twist not only tantalizes the taste buds but also ensures a spectrum of nutrients, embodying the spirit of adaptability in the face of a globalized culinary landscape.

A pivotal aspect of the balance between tradition and modernity lies in the mindful incorporation of technology. From apps that track nutritional intake to wearable devices that monitor physical activity, technology has become an ally in our quest for optimal health. The integration of science-backed information empowers individuals to make informed choices, bridging the gap between ancient wisdom and contemporary knowledge.

In essence, the art of balancing traditional and contemporary dietary principles is a dynamic dance, a synthesis of the timeless and the avant-garde. It invites us to honor the ancestral wisdom that has withstood the test of time while embracing the innovative tools that enhance our understanding of nutrition. In this delicate equilibrium, we find a roadmap to sustained well-being – a journey where the roots of tradition anchor us, and the wings of innovation propel us toward a future where health is a harmonious marriage of the old and the new.

3.2 Superfoods and their impact on vitality:

In the kaleidoscope of nutrition, certain foods stand out as veritable powerhouses, often earning the title of "superfoods" for their exceptional nutrient density and potential impact on vitality. These nutritional juggernauts, packed with a myriad of essential vitamins, minerals, antioxidants, and other bioactive compounds, play a pivotal role in enhancing overall well-being and vitality.

1. Berries:

Berries, such as blueberries, strawberries, and raspberries, are rich in antioxidants, particularly anthocyanins. These compounds have been linked to improved cognitive function, reduced inflammation, and a bolstered immune system, contributing to sustained vitality.

2. Leafy Greens:

Dark, leafy greens like kale, spinach, and Swiss chard are nutrient powerhouses, providing an abundance of vitamins, minerals, and phytochemicals. Their high folate content supports energy metabolism, while antioxidants combat oxidative stress, fostering vitality at the cellular level.

3. Fatty Fish:

Fatty fish like salmon, mackerel, and sardines are brimming with omega-3 fatty acids. These essential fats support heart health, reduce inflammation, and may positively influence mood and cognitive function, contributing to an overall sense of vitality.

4. Nuts and Seeds:

Almonds, walnuts, chia seeds, and flaxseeds are nutrient-dense options rich in healthy fats, fiber, and various vitamins and minerals. These foods provide sustained energy, support cardiovascular health, and contribute to overall vitality.

5. Turmeric:

Turmeric contains curcumin, a potent anti-inflammatory compound with antioxidant properties. Studies suggest that curcumin may help alleviate symptoms associated with chronic inflammation, promoting joint health and overall vitality.

6. Green Tea:

Green tea is renowned for its high concentration of catechins, potent antioxidants that may have a range of health benefits. These include improved cognitive function, enhanced metabolism, and potential protection against age-related decline, contributing to sustained vitality.

7. Greek Yogurt:

Greek yogurt is a rich source of protein, probiotics, and essential nutrients like calcium. The combination of protein and probiotics supports digestive health, immune function, and muscle maintenance, contributing to an overall sense of vitality.

8. Quinoa:

Quinoa is a nutrient-dense whole grain, providing a complete protein source along with essential vitamins and minerals. Its complex carbohydrates release energy slowly, promoting stable blood sugar levels and sustained vitality.

9. Dark Chocolate:

Dark chocolate, in moderation, is rich in flavonoids and antioxidants. Consuming high-quality dark chocolate has been associated with improved mood, enhanced cognitive function, and potential cardiovascular benefits, contributing to overall vitality.

10. Avocado:

Avocado is a nutrient-dense fruit loaded with healthy monounsaturated fats, vitamins, and minerals. These fats support heart health, and the diverse array of nutrients contributes to sustained energy and vitality.

Including a range of superfoods in a diet that is well-balanced can be a key component in fostering vitality. To achieve and sustain optimal vitality, it is imperative to prioritize general dietary patterns and lifestyle factors, understanding that a comprehensive approach to nutrition, exercise, sleep, and stress management is necessary.

CHAPTER 4: INTEGRATING ANCIENT PRACTICES

The notion of Renaissance Fitness emerges as a light in the enthralling fabric of human experience, weaving together the threads of ancient knowledge and modern desires. It is a symphony that harmonizes old well-being traditions with the vibrant pulse of the modern day, a celebration of the everlasting dance between tradition and innovation.

The echoes of old techniques resound strongly as we start on the road of self-discovery and physical empowerment. Our forefathers, astute keepers of health and vigor, bequeathed us a treasure mine of wisdom rooted in traditions that have stood the test of time. The Renaissance Fitness paradigm urges us to dust off these old manuscripts and integrate them into the fabric of our modern lives with reverence.

Picture a mosaic where the meditative stillness of yoga meets the vibrant cadence of high-intensity interval training; where the fluidity of Tai Chi gracefully waltzes with the precision of weightlifting. In the crucible of Renaissance Fitness, the alchemy of diverse disciplines converges, forging a path to unleash our full physical potential.

At its core, Renaissance Fitness is a testament to the adaptability of the human spirit and the symbiotic relationship between tradition and progress. It beckons us to explore the labyrinth of ancient practices, unlocking the secrets of longevity, strength, and holistic well-being. From the yogic serenity that centers the mind to the disciplined artistry of martial traditions sculpting the body, each ancient practice is a brushstroke in the masterpiece of our fitness journey.

In this modern age, where the relentless pace of life often threatens to sever our connection with our physical selves, Renaissance Fitness becomes a sanctuary. It is a sanctuary where the echoes of ancient breath control techniques guide us through the cacophony of stress, where the rhythm of primal movement patterns rekindles the innate wisdom of our bodies.

The Renaissance Fitness philosophy is a bridge across time, inviting us to traverse the chasm between the ancients and the contemporary. It encourages us to honor the wisdom of our forebears while fearlessly embracing the cutting-edge innovations that science and technology offer. It is a synthesis that propels us towards a future where the ancient and the modern coalesce, not in contradiction, but in a harmonious celebration of human potential.

As we embark on the transformative journey of Renaissance Fitness, let us be mindful of the profound interplay between the roots of tradition and the shoots of innovation. In each rep, in each stretch, and in every meditative pause, we find the alchemical blend of ancient practices and modern methodologies, unlocking the gates to a realm where our physical prowess, mental clarity, and spiritual well-being converge.

May the Renaissance Fitness revolution be a celebration of unity—a fusion of time-honored principles and contemporary insights, guiding us towards a holistic embodiment of our truest, most vibrant selves in the mosaic of existence.

4.1 Yoga, tai chi, and other timeless disciplines:

Yoga, Tai Chi, and a myriad of other timeless disciplines stand as ancient sentinels, guardians of well-being, and wisdom, inviting us to embark on a profound journey of self-discovery and holistic flourishing.

Yoga, with its roots reaching deep into the spiritual soil of ancient India, is a transcendent practice that seamlessly weaves the tapestry of physical postures, breath control, and meditation. It is a sacred dance of the body and mind, a harmonious symphony that seeks to unite the individual with the universal. Through the gentle arcs of asanas and the serene flow of pranayama, yoga whispers to the soul, unraveling layers of tension and ushering in a tranquil balance.

Tai Chi, a graceful martial art born from the ancient Chinese philosophies of Taoism and Confucianism, is a poetic expression of balance and energy. Its slow, deliberate movements, akin to a soft ballet, invite practitioners into a state of mindfulness and meditation in motion. In the mesmerizing dance of Tai Chi, the body becomes a vessel for the ebb and flow of chi, the life force that animates the universe, fostering a sense of internal harmony and external grace.

Beyond these luminaries, there exists a constellation of other timeless disciplines that have traversed the corridors of history to reach us. Pilates, with its focus on core strength and flexibility, draws inspiration from the teachings of Joseph Pilates, intertwining the physical and the mental. Martial arts, spanning a rich spectrum from Karate to Kung Fu, embody the disciplined path of warriors, offering not just physical prowess but also instilling virtues of honor, respect, and self-control.

As we embrace these timeless disciplines in the modern age, they become not relics of a bygone era, but living traditions that bridge the gap between antiquity and innovation. In the hustle and bustle of the contemporary world, where the digital heartbeat races, these ancient practices emerge as sanctuaries—places where the clamor of the external world is hushed, and individuals can reconnect with the ancient rhythms of their own bodies and minds.

The essence of these disciplines lies not merely in the physical postures or sequences but in the mindful intention that accompanies each movement. They are gateways to a deeper understanding of oneself, offering a sacred space for introspection, introspection, and self-realization. In the seamless marriage of body and spirit, they transcend the confines of mere exercise, evolving into transformative tools that illuminate the path to holistic well-being.

As we weave the threads of Yoga, Tai Chi, and other timeless disciplines into the fabric of our lives, let us embrace the wisdom of the ancients with gratitude. In doing so, we honor not only the rich tapestry of human heritage but also set forth on a journey of personal enlightenment—a journey where the whispers of the past guide us toward a harmonious existence in the ever-evolving dance of the present.

4.2 Adapting ancient wisdom to modern lifestyles:

In the fast-paced, digitally-driven landscape of the modern world, the integration of ancient wisdom into our lifestyles becomes a poignant endeavor—a quest to harmonize the timeless with the contemporary, fostering a holistic approach to well-being.

The venerable teachings of ancient wisdom, rooted in cultures across the globe, serve as guiding stars in our quest for balance, purpose, and inner peace. As we adapt these age-old principles to the exigencies of our daily lives, we embark on a transformative journey, forging a path that bridges antiquity with innovation.

One of the cornerstones of this adaptation is mindfulness—an ancient practice that finds newfound relevance in the tumultuous currents of our present existence. The art of being fully present in the moment, cultivated through meditation and conscious awareness, becomes a powerful antidote to the digital distractions that threaten to pull us away from the richness of our lives. In the relentless pursuit of productivity, mindfulness emerges as a beacon, reminding us to savor the nuances of each experience and cultivate a sense of inner calm amidst the chaos.

Ancient dietary wisdom, deeply rooted in traditions such as Ayurveda and traditional Chinese medicine, offers a compass to navigate the labyrinth of modern nutrition. The emphasis on whole, unprocessed foods, mindful eating, and the recognition of the interconnectedness between diet and well-being becomes a timeless roadmap for fostering optimal health. Integrating these principles into our dietary choices allows us to not only fuel our bodies but also nourish our spirits, fostering a harmonious relationship with the sustenance that nature provides.

In the realm of movement, the fusion of ancient practices like Yoga and Tai Chi with contemporary exercise modalities yields a holistic approach to physical well-being. Yoga, with its emphasis on flexibility, strength, and breath control, becomes a sanctuary for those seeking respite from sedentary lifestyles. Tai Chi, with its gentle, flowing movements, serves as a counterbalance to the high-impact nature of modern workouts, offering a pathway to longevity and grace in motion.

Furthermore, the art of slowing down, a timeless wisdom found in ancient philosophies, becomes a revolutionary act in the context of our modern rush. From the ancient Japanese practice of forest bathing to the contemplative traditions of Stoicism, the invitation to pause, reflect, and connect with the natural rhythms of life becomes a balm for the weary soul. Embracing moments of stillness in our hyperactive lives becomes a deliberate choice—an homage to the ancient understanding that true wisdom often unfolds in the spaces between breaths.

As we navigate the currents of the 21st century, adapting ancient wisdom to modern lifestyles is not a nostalgic reverie but a vital necessity. It is an admission that the deep truths our ancestors found still serve as enduring lights in the middle of fast progress and modern conveniences. Not only do we find a way to well-being by incorporating the timeless wisdom of humanity's journey into our lives, but we also build a bridge to connect with it.

CHAPTER 5: TECH-ASSISTED WELLNESS

The birth of the modern age has brought about a paradigm change in the way we see and pursue well-being in the broad fabric of human existence. In this day and age of limitless technology developments, a profound confluence of cutting-edge innovation and holistic well-being has given rise to what may properly be called "Renaissance Fitness." This revolutionary approach to wellness goes beyond conventional bounds, enabling people to go on a journey of self-discovery, empowerment, and optimization.

At the heart of Renaissance Fitness lies a harmonious blend of age-old wisdom and contemporary technological prowess. It is a celebration of the human spirit's unyielding quest for improvement, facilitated and enhanced by the limitless possibilities offered by modern technology. In a world where the pace of life seems to quicken with each passing day, Renaissance Fitness serves as a beacon, guiding individuals toward unlocking their true potential in the most profound and holistic manner.

Technology, once viewed as a mere tool, has evolved into a benevolent companion on the path to wellness. From wearable fitness trackers that meticulously monitor every heartbeat to virtual reality experiences that transport us to realms of tranquility, technology now stands as a silent ally, empowering us to make informed decisions about our health and well-being. It is the bridge that connects the ancient wisdom of mindful living with the precision of data-driven insights, offering a nuanced understanding of our bodies, minds, and overall wellness.

Personalized well-being takes center stage at Renaissance Fitness. Individuals are no longer limited to generic fitness regimes; instead, they may adapt their well-being journey to their specific requirements, interests, and objectives. Artificial intelligence algorithms, data analytics, and smart devices work together to create personalized wellness regimens, ensuring that each step toward fitness is a deliberate step toward personal perfection.

The Renaissance Fitness philosophy extends beyond the physical realm, recognizing the intricate interplay between mental and emotional well-being. Meditation apps, guided mindfulness sessions, and biofeedback technologies seamlessly integrate into the fabric of daily life, fostering a holistic approach to wellness that acknowledges the interconnectedness of mind, body, and spirit. The modern age, with all its complexities, becomes a canvas upon which individuals paint their own masterpieces of vitality and fulfillment.

As we accept the Renaissance Fitness paradigm, the basic idea of what it means to be fit changes dramatically. It goes beyond the surface measures of weight and appearance to explore resilience, balance, and long-term vitality. It is an invitation to mold not only the body, but also a life full of meaning, joy, and resilience.

Finally, Renaissance Fitness exemplifies the astonishing synergy between humanity's ageless desire for well-being and the technical wonders that define our modern civilization. It is an homage to the tenacious human spirit, which is always growing and adapting to change. So, join me on this transforming trip where technology and wellness collide and the Renaissance Fitness unfolds, unveiling huge landscapes of our untapped potential in the contemporary day.

5.1 Wearables and smart devices for fitness tracking:

Wearables and smart gadgets have emerged as indispensable partners on the route to optimal health in the changing environment of modern wellness. These technical marvels, outfitted with a plethora of sensors and innovative technologies, enable people to monitor, evaluate, and improve many aspects of their physical well-being. Here, we dig into the transformational world of wearables and smart gadgets for fitness tracking, investigating how they are changing our approach to health.

1. Wearable Fitness Trackers:

These little, wrist-worn gadgets have become associated with the arsenal of the modern exercise fanatic. They are packed with sensors like accelerometers, gyroscopes, and heart rate monitors that precisely record data on steps taken, distance traveled, calories expended, and even sleep habits.

Furthermore, many modern trackers offer real-time feedback and notifications, encouraging users to stay active throughout the day. The seamless integration of these wearables into daily life fosters a heightened awareness of one's physical activity, promoting a more active and health-conscious lifestyle.

2. Smartwatches:

The convergence of fitness tracking and smartwatch technology has given rise to a versatile device that transcends traditional boundaries. Smartwatches not only monitor physical activity but also serve as extensions of smartphones, offering features like call notifications, messaging, and even app integrations.

With GPS capabilities, smartwatches enable accurate tracking of outdoor activities such as running and cycling. They have become indispensable tools for individuals seeking a holistic approach to health, seamlessly integrating fitness tracking with the demands of modern life.

3. Biometric Sensors:

Beyond the realm of step counts and calories, wearable devices now incorporate advanced biometric sensors to provide a more comprehensive understanding of one's health. These sensors can measure vital signs such as heart rate variability, skin temperature, and even blood oxygen levels.

The availability of this nuanced data empowers users to gain insights into their overall well-being, facilitating informed decisions about training intensity, recovery, and stress management.

4. Smart Clothing:

Innovations in textile technology have given rise to smart clothing embedded with sensors that capture a wealth of physiological data. From shirts that monitor heart rate to socks that analyze gait, these garments offer a non-intrusive way to gather information about various aspects of physical performance.

The incorporation of sensors into clothes eliminates the need for extra equipment, resulting in a discrete and comfortable solution for continuous fitness tracking.

5. Fitness Apps and Ecosystems:

The synergy between wearable devices and fitness apps creates a robust ecosystem for users to set goals, track progress, and receive personalized insights. These apps often leverage artificial intelligence to analyze data and provide actionable recommendations, creating a tailored approach to fitness.

Integration with social platforms allows users to share achievements, fostering a sense of community and motivation. This interconnected web of technology transforms fitness from a solitary endeavor into a collaborative and empowering experience.

In the era of wearables and smart devices, the marriage of technology and fitness has ushered in a new era of personalized well-being. As these devices continue to evolve, they not only track our physical activity but also inspire us to unleash our potential, fostering a proactive and empowered approach to health in the modern age.

5.2 Apps and tools for personalized wellness plans:

In the age of personalized wellness, a plethora of apps and tools have emerged, harnessing the power of technology to tailor health and well-being plans to individual needs. These innovative solutions go beyond generic approaches, offering users a personalized and data-driven journey toward optimal health. Here, we explore a selection of apps and tools that exemplify the transformative landscape of personalized wellness plans:

1. MyFitnessPal:

MyFitnessPal is a comprehensive app that facilitates personalized wellness plans by integrating fitness tracking with nutrition monitoring. Users can log their meals, track calories, set fitness goals, and access a vast database of foods. The app's ability to sync with various wearables and other fitness apps enhances its utility, creating a seamless experience for users aiming to achieve their unique health objectives.

2. Fitbit:

Fitbit, renowned for its wearable devices, offers an app that extends the fitness tracking experience. The app not only captures physical activity data but also provides insights into sleep patterns, heart rate, and more. Fitbit's personalized guidance, based on user data, helps individuals set achievable goals and adapt their wellness plans to their evolving needs.

3. Headspace:

Mental well-being is a crucial component of personalized wellness, and Headspace specializes in mindfulness and meditation. The app offers guided meditation sessions, sleep exercises, and mindful living courses. With personalized recommendations based on user preferences and goals, Headspace fosters a holistic approach to wellness that encompasses both body and mind.

4. Nike Training Club:

The Nike Training Club app stands out for individuals looking for individualized fitness programs. It customizes workouts depending on your fitness level, goals, and time constraints. The adaptive elements of the software improve in response to the user's success, ensuring that the exercise regimen remains tough and effective. Professional trainers' video advice adds an interactive element to the experience.

5. 8fit:

8fit combines personalized fitness and nutrition plans in a user-friendly app. Users begin by providing information about their fitness goals, dietary preferences, and current fitness levels. The app then crafts a customized plan, offering workout routines and meal suggestions. Regular progress tracking ensures that the plan adapts to the user's changing needs.

6. Lifesum:

Lifesum is a versatile app that combines diet tracking with personalized meal plans. It considers dietary preferences, health goals, and lifestyle factors to create tailored meal suggestions. The app's integration with wearables and fitness trackers allows for a comprehensive overview of the user's health and wellness journey.

7. CARROT Wellness:

CARROT Wellness adds a unique, gamified twist to personalized wellness plans. The app leverages humor and rewards to motivate users to achieve their fitness goals. Through personalized challenges and dynamic feedback, CARROT Wellness turns wellness into an engaging and entertaining experience.

8. Habitica:

Habitica transforms personal development into a game, where users create avatars and gain rewards for completing wellness-related tasks. This app gamifies goal-setting, making it an engaging tool for individuals looking to establish and maintain healthy habits.

In the field of customized wellness, these applications and tools combine user data, cutting-edge technology, and professional advice. Individuals who embrace these solutions can begin on a path that goes beyond one-size-fits-all methods, unlocking the possibility for long-term well-being suited to their specific requirements and objectives.

CHAPTER 6: MIND-BODY CONNECTION

A profound and sophisticated dance exists in the fabric of human existence between the ethereal world of the mind and the physical refuge of the body. This interaction, this cosmic synergy, is what gives rise to the Mind-Body Connection—a concept that transcends time and finds echo in the very fabric of our existence. Within this link, a beacon of enlightenment develops, a guiding light that guides us through the maze of our own potential—this is Renaissance Fitness: Unleashing Your Potential in the Modern Age.

In the grand tapestry of history, the Renaissance was an epoch that witnessed the blossoming of human intellect and creativity. Fast forward to the present day, and we find ourselves at the dawn of a new era—a modern renaissance, where the pursuit of physical and mental excellence takes center stage. Renaissance Fitness, then, becomes not merely a regimen of exercise but a holistic philosophy that seeks to harmonize the intricate symphony of mind and body.

At its core, Renaissance Fitness beckons us to rediscover the profound connection between the cerebral and corporeal realms. It is an invitation to embark on a journey of self-discovery, where the contours of the mind echo in the sinews of the body, and vice versa. The pulsating heartbeat of each workout becomes a rhythmic meditation, a communion between mental fortitude and physical resilience.

In the cacophony of the modern age, where the ceaseless demands of life threaten to disentangle our thoughts and fragment our bodies, Renaissance Fitness emerges as a sanctuary—an oasis of balance. It is not a mere pursuit of sculpted physiques but a quest for a harmonious existence, where mental acuity and physical vitality converge in a seamless dance.

Through the disciplined cadence of exercise, the mind finds solace in the present moment. In the repetition of each movement, the chaos of daily life dissipates, and a serene clarity takes root. Renaissance Fitness, in its essence, becomes a meditative practice, a mindful journey that transforms the sweat of exertion into the elixir of mental tranquility.

Simultaneously, as the body undergoes the crucible of physical exertion, the mind too experiences a metamorphosis. It learns the language of resilience, resilience that echoes in the reverberations of muscles pushed to their limits. In the crucible of the gym or the open expanse of nature, the mind forges its own Renaissance—a rebirth of determination, willpower, and an unwavering belief in one's own potential.

This modern-day Renaissance Fitness is not limited to the gym; it pervades all aspects of our lives. It is a way of life, a philosophy that promotes the benefits of holistic well-being. It inspires us to be masters of our own fate, both intellectually and physically. In this quest, the mind and body cease to be separate entities and instead become co-authors of a story, a story that unfolds with every conscious breath and purposeful action.

As we navigate the uncharted waters of the modern age, let Renaissance Fitness be our compass—a compass that guides us to the shores of self-realization, where the mind and body converge to unleash the latent potential within. It is a celebration of the human spirit, a testament to our ability to transcend the ordinary and embrace the extraordinary. In the mosaic of our existence, let Renaissance Fitness be the vibrant brushstroke that paints a masterpiece of vitality, resilience, and unparalleled self-discovery.

6.1 The role of mental well-being in physical fitness:

The interplay between mental well-being and physical fitness forms a dynamic and symbiotic relationship that significantly influences overall health. Beyond the surface level of muscles and cardiovascular endurance, the state of one's mental health is a powerful determinant of physical well-being. This intricate connection underscores the importance of understanding and nurturing both aspects for a holistic approach to health and fitness.

1. Motivation and Consistency:

Mental well-being serves as the bedrock of motivation. A positive mental state fosters the drive to engage in physical activities consistently. When individuals are mentally resilient and focused, they are more likely to adhere to workout routines, make healthier lifestyle choices, and persevere through challenges. Conversely, mental health struggles may lead to a lack of motivation, hindering adherence to fitness regimens.

2. Stress Management:

Physical activity is a potent stress reliever, and mental well-being plays a pivotal role in stress management. Chronic stress can manifest physically, affecting the body's hormonal balance and potentially impeding fitness progress. Regular exercise, fueled by positive mental health, becomes a dual-purpose remedy—alleviating stress and contributing to physical fitness.

3. Cognitive Function and Coordination:

Mental clarity and cognitive function are integral to physical fitness. A healthy mind enhances coordination, concentration, and the ability to perform exercises with precision. Conversely, conditions affecting mental well-being, such as anxiety or depression, may impact coordination and focus during workouts, potentially compromising the effectiveness of physical activities.

4. Quality of Workouts:

The mindset one brings to a workout significantly influences its quality. A positive mental state fosters enthusiasm, determination, and the ability to push physical boundaries. Conversely, mental fatigue or negative thoughts can lead to suboptimal workouts. Therefore, mental well-being contributes to the efficacy of exercise sessions and the achievement of fitness goals.

5. Recovery and Sleep:

Adequate rest and recovery are essential components of any fitness regimen. Mental well-being directly affects sleep quality and the body's ability to recover from physical exertion. Conditions like insomnia or heightened stress levels can hinder recovery, potentially impeding progress and increasing the risk of injuries.

6. Hormonal Balance:

Mental well-being influences the body's hormonal balance. Stress, anxiety, or depression can disrupt hormone levels, impacting metabolism, muscle growth, and overall physical health. Engaging in activities that promote mental well-being, such as mindfulness or relaxation techniques, contributes to hormonal equilibrium and supports physical fitness.

7. Lifestyle Choices:

Mental health influences lifestyle choices that can either support or undermine physical fitness. Individuals with positive mental well-being are more likely to make healthy dietary choices, avoid harmful habits, and engage in activities that promote overall well-being. Conversely, mental health challenges may lead to sedentary behavior, poor nutrition, or other habits detrimental to physical health.

Recognizing the intricate link between mental well-being and physical fitness is paramount for achieving a balanced and sustainable approach to health. Embracing strategies that address both aspects—such as mindfulness practices, stress-reducing activities, and seeking professional support when needed—can pave the way for a more resilient, motivated, and ultimately healthier self.

6.2 Mindfulness and stress management for overall health:

Mindfulness and stress management are powerful tools that contribute significantly to overall health and well-being. In a world marked by constant stimuli and demands, incorporating mindfulness practices into daily life can be transformative, providing a holistic approach to stress reduction and enhancing various aspects of one's health. Here's a closer look at how mindfulness and stress management contribute to overall well-being:

1. Stress Reduction:

Mindfulness involves being fully present in the current moment without judgment. Through practices such as meditation, deep breathing, or mindful awareness, individuals can cultivate a heightened sense of awareness that counteracts the detrimental effects of chronic stress. Mindfulness has been shown to lower cortisol levels, reducing the physiological impact of stress on the body.

2. Emotional Regulation:

Mindfulness allows individuals to observe their thoughts and emotions without being overwhelmed by them. This heightened self-awareness fosters emotional regulation, empowering individuals to respond to stressors in a calm and composed manner. By developing a non-reactive mindset, individuals can navigate challenges with greater resilience and maintain emotional equilibrium.

3. Improved Mental Health:

Regular mindfulness practice has been associated with reduced symptoms of anxiety, depression, and other mental health conditions. By promoting a positive and non-judgmental attitude towards one's thoughts and experiences, mindfulness contributes to a healthier mental state, fostering a sense of calm and inner peace.

4. Enhanced Cognitive Function:

Mindfulness practices have been linked to improvements in cognitive function, including attention, memory, and problem-solving skills. By training the mind to focus on the present moment, individuals can enhance their cognitive abilities, leading to increased mental clarity and effectiveness in daily tasks.

5. Better Sleep Quality:

Mindfulness meditation and relaxation techniques are effective in promoting better sleep quality. By reducing stress and calming the mind, individuals can overcome insomnia or sleep disturbances. Improved sleep not only contributes to overall well-being but also supports physical health and immune function.

6. Lower Blood Pressure:

Chronic stress is a known contributor to elevated blood pressure, increasing the risk of cardiovascular issues. Mindfulness practices, through their stress-reducing effects, have been associated with lower blood pressure levels. This, in turn, contributes to cardiovascular health and reduces the risk of related conditions.

7. Enhanced Self-Awareness:

Mindfulness encourages self-reflection and self-awareness. By becoming attuned to one's thoughts, feelings, and bodily sensations, individuals can identify sources of stress and understand their reactions to various situations. This heightened self-awareness empowers individuals to make conscious choices that align with their well-being.

8. Improved Immune Function:

Chronic stress can weaken the immune system, making individuals more susceptible to illness. Mindfulness practices have been linked to improvements in immune function, promoting a healthier and more robust defense against infections and diseases.

9. Long-Term Well-Being:

Incorporating mindfulness into daily life fosters a mindset that extends beyond immediate stressors. It encourages individuals to embrace a more mindful approach to living, making choices that prioritize overall well-being in the long term.

Incorporating mindfulness practices, such as meditation, mindful breathing, or yoga, into a daily routine can be a valuable investment in overall health. By cultivating a present-moment awareness and adopting effective stress management strategies, individuals can enhance their resilience, emotional well-being, and overall quality of life.

CHAPTER 7: FUNCTIONAL FITNESS FOR EVERYDAY LIFE

Functional fitness is a holistic approach to exercise that focuses on enhancing overall physical function, mobility, and strength to improve one's ability to perform daily activities effectively and safely. Unlike traditional fitness routines that may isolate muscle groups, functional fitness incorporates movements that mimic real-life activities, making it particularly relevant for enhancing everyday life. Here are the key principles and benefits of functional fitness:

1. Multidimensional Movements:
Functional fitness emphasizes multi-joint movements that engage multiple muscle groups simultaneously. Exercises often involve pushing, pulling, twisting, bending, and lifting, mirroring the diverse actions performed in daily life.

2. Core Stability:

Core strength is a foundational aspect of functional fitness. A strong core provides stability for various movements, supports proper posture, and helps prevent injuries during activities like lifting, bending, and reaching.

3. Real-Life Applications:

Exercises in functional fitness are designed to improve performance in everyday tasks. This includes activities like carrying groceries, lifting children, reaching for items on high shelves, and maintaining balance during daily movements.

4. Balance and Coordination:

Functional fitness workouts often include exercises that challenge balance and coordination. Enhancing these skills is crucial for preventing falls and improving overall stability in various situations.

5. Adaptability:

Functional fitness routines can be adapted to suit individual fitness levels, making them accessible for people of all ages and abilities. Whether you're a seasoned athlete or a beginner, functional exercises can be modified to accommodate your current fitness level.

6. Incorporation of Body Weight:

Many functional exercises use body weight as resistance, reducing the need for specialized equipment. This makes functional fitness convenient for individuals who prefer home workouts or have limited access to gym equipment.

7. Improved Joint Mobility:

Functional movements often involve a full range of motion, promoting joint flexibility and mobility. This is particularly beneficial for maintaining joint health and preventing stiffness associated with sedentary lifestyles.

8. Time Efficiency:

Functional workouts can be time-efficient, as they often engage multiple muscle groups simultaneously. This is advantageous for individuals with busy schedules, allowing them to achieve effective workouts in shorter durations.

9. Injury Prevention:

By focusing on functional movements and addressing imbalances in strength and flexibility, functional fitness helps reduce the risk of injuries both during workouts and in everyday activities.

10. Enhanced Quality of Life:

Ultimately, the goal of functional fitness is to enhance the quality of life by improving one's ability to move with ease and confidence. Whether it's participating in recreational activities, playing with children, or maintaining independence as we age, functional fitness contributes to a more fulfilling and active lifestyle.

Incorporating functional fitness into your routine can be achieved through a variety of exercises such as squats, lunges, planks, and functional training equipment like resistance bands, kettlebells, and stability balls. As with any exercise program, it's advisable to consult with a fitness professional or healthcare provider, especially if you have pre-existing health conditions or concerns.

7.1 Building strength and mobility for real-world scenarios:

In the labyrinth of our daily lives, where unpredictability reigns and challenges manifest in myriad forms, the importance of cultivating strength and mobility transcends the confines of traditional exercise routines. It is a call to arms, an acknowledgment that the gym is but a microcosm of the vast and dynamic landscapes we navigate daily. Building strength and mobility for real-world scenarios is not just a fitness pursuit; it is a commitment to fortifying ourselves for the unpredictable journey that is life.

Imagine a scenario where the demands of the day require more than the ability to lift heavy weights in a controlled environment. Consider the need to carry groceries up flights of stairs, to chase after a bus, or to bend and twist to pick up a fallen object. These are the moments where functional strength, born from exercises that mimic real-life movements, emerges as a formidable ally.

Functional strength is the key that unlocks doors in the real world. It is the strength to push, pull, lift, and carry, seamlessly translating into everyday tasks. Whether it's moving furniture, playing with children, or simply maintaining balance on uneven terrain, a foundation of functional strength equips us to handle the physical demands of life's unpredictable choreography.

Yet, strength alone is but one facet of the multifaceted jewel that is real-world preparedness. Mobility, the often-overlooked sibling of strength, is equally indispensable. It is the ability to move with purpose and precision, to navigate a world that requires flexibility and adaptability. In the dance of life, where every step may present a new challenge, mobility is the choreography that allows us to move with grace and confidence.

Consider the significance of a mobile spine that twists and turns effortlessly, or shoulders that can reach, lift, and carry without constraint. In the real world, where movement is multidirectional and unpredictable, mobility becomes the silent partner of strength, ensuring that our bodies can respond to the ever-changing demands of our environment.

The amalgamation of strength and mobility is not a mere physical endeavor; it is a holistic approach to well-being. As we cultivate physical resilience, we simultaneously nurture mental fortitude. The confidence gained from knowing that our bodies are capable of meeting real-world challenges head-on permeates into our psyche, fostering a mindset that embraces obstacles as opportunities for growth.

The journey towards building strength and mobility for real-world scenarios is not a solitary trek. It is a shared exploration, a communal pursuit that finds its roots in the recognition that we are all navigating the same unpredictable terrain. In fitness communities, the exchange of knowledge, support, and encouragement becomes the compass guiding individuals toward their collective goal of functional prowess.

In conclusion, the quest for strength and mobility is not confined to the walls of a gym but extends into the vast expanse of our daily lives. It is a journey marked by functional movements, real-world applications, and a holistic understanding of well-being. As we forge ahead, may we cultivate strength and mobility not only for the sake of physical prowess but as a testament to our resilience in the face of life's unpredictable tapestry.

7.2 Practical exercises for functional fitness:

Functional fitness revolves around exercises that mimic and enhance the movements we perform in our everyday lives. These exercises target multiple muscle groups, improve coordination, and increase overall mobility. Here are some practical exercises for functional fitness:

1. Squat:

*Stand with feet shoulder-width apart.

*Lower your body as if sitting back into a chair, keeping your back straight.

*Rise back up to the starting position.

*This exercise mimics the motion of sitting and standing, essential for daily activities.

2. Lunges:

*Take a step forward with one foot and lower your body until both knees are bent at a 90-degree angle.

*Push back to the starting position and repeat on the other leg.

*Lunges improve balance and mimic walking or climbing stairs.

3. Deadlift:

*Stand with feet hip-width apart, holding a weight in front of you.

*Hinge at the hips and lower the weight towards the ground while keeping your back straight.

*Return to the upright position.

*This exercise mimics lifting objects from the ground, promoting a strong and stable lower back.

4. Push-ups:

*Start in a plank position with hands shoulder-width apart.

*Lower your body by bending your elbows, then push back up to the starting position.

*Push-ups strengthen the chest, shoulders, and core, essential for various pushing movements in daily life.

5. Pull-ups:

*Use a pull-up bar or sturdy surface.

*Hang from the bar and pull your body upward until your chin is above the bar.

*Lower yourself back down.

*Pull-ups target the upper body, specifically the back and arms, supporting activities like lifting or pulling.

6. Plank:

*Begin in a push-up position, then lower onto your forearms.
*Keep your body in a straight line from head to heels.
*Hold the position for as long as possible.
*Planks engage the core and promote stability, crucial for various movements and activities.

7. Farmers' Walk:

*Hold a heavy weight (dumbbells or kettlebells) in each hand.
*Walk a set distance maintaining an upright posture.
*Farmers' walks enhance grip strength, and core stability, and simulate carrying groceries or other heavy items.

8. Medicine Ball Throws:

*Stand with feet shoulder-width apart, holding a medicine ball.
*Explosively throw the ball against a wall or to a partner.
*This exercise improves power and coordination, resembling movements like tossing or lifting objects.

9. Step-Ups:

*Use a sturdy platform or step.

*Step up with one foot and bring the other knee toward your chest.

*Step back down and repeat on the other leg.

*Step-ups simulate climbing stairs and enhance lower body strength.

10. Turkish Get-Up:

*Lie on your back holding a kettlebell.

*Perform a series of movements to stand up, then reverse the process to return to the starting position.

*The Turkish Get-Up promotes total-body strength, stability, and mobility.

If you're new to these workouts or have any current health problems, always use good form and check with a fitness professional. As your strength and fitness levels improve, gradually increase the intensity and volume.

CHAPTER 8: SLEEP SCIENCE AND RECOVERY

There's a deep tapestry of renewal and vitality woven through the complex dance of mind, body, and spirit where holistic well-being is concerned. The field that goes beyond the norm, where the alchemy of recovery and sleep science creates a symphony of rebirth, is at the center of this elaborate design. A light shines on the path toward Renaissance Fitness, an era in which our hidden potential is not only acknowledged but also unlocked with unmatched grace, as we set out on the path of self-discovery in the modern era.

In the cadence of our hectic lives, where the pulsating rhythm of daily demands often drowns the melody of tranquility, the significance of sleep science becomes an anthem for the rejuvenation of our very essence. It is not merely the act of closing our eyes and succumbing to the embrace of night; it is an art, a delicate ballet choreographed by the circadian rhythms that govern our internal symphony. Renaissance Fitness, in its essence, heralds an era where the understanding of sleep transcends the realm of mere rest and delves into the intricate nuances of recovery.

In the crucible of the modern age, where technology and progress propel us forward, the principles of Renaissance Fitness offer a sanctuary—a sacred space where the rejuvenation of mind and body becomes a sacred ritual. It is here that we unfurl the canvas of sleep science, exploring the intricate brushstrokes that paint a portrait of holistic well-being. From the microcosmic dance of neurotransmitters to the macrocosmic journey of REM cycles, each nuance becomes a stroke in the masterpiece of our vitality.

As we traverse the landscape of Renaissance Fitness, the canvas extends beyond the sanctity of sleep to embrace the symphony of recovery. It is a testament to the resilience of the human spirit, an acknowledgment that the ebb and flow of life require moments of reprieve and renewal. Recovery becomes the nurturing touch, the unseen hands that mend the tapestry of our existence, ensuring that each thread, no matter how delicate, contributes to the strength of the whole.

In the crucible of Renaissance Fitness, we discover that recovery is not synonymous with idleness, but rather a dynamic interplay between activity and repose. It is a conscious dance with the rhythms of restoration—a nuanced choreography that acknowledges the varied needs of our physical, mental, and emotional selves. From the meditative cadence of mindful movement to the therapeutic embrace of stillness, recovery becomes an integral note in the symphony of our existence.

As we delve deeper into the sanctuary of Renaissance Fitness, we unveil the transformative power embedded in the fusion of sleep science and recovery. It is a harmonious marriage where the alchemical process of rejuvenation unfolds, ushering us into a realm where the boundaries between our dormant potential and realized capabilities blur. It is an invitation to embrace the subtleties of our inner landscape, to honor the wisdom encoded in the whispers of our bodies and minds.

Renaissance Fitness arises as a monument to the artistry of self-care in the fabric of life, where the warp and weft of existence intertwine. We start on a trip that transcends the commonplace via the gateway of sleep science and recovery, ushering in an era in which our latent potential is set free to dance with the rhythms of our most true selves. It's an homage to the human spirit, a song that echoes through the hallways of the contemporary day with the symphony of rejuvenation.

8.1 Optimizing sleep for physical and mental recovery:

Optimizing sleep for both physical and mental recovery is a cornerstone of overall well-being. The profound impact of quality sleep on our body and mind cannot be overstated, as it serves as a critical catalyst for optimal functioning, resilience, and vitality. Here are key principles to consider in the quest to maximize the rejuvenating potential of your sleep:

1. Prioritize Consistent Sleep Schedule:

Establish a regular sleep-wake cycle by going to bed and waking up at the same time every day, even on weekends. This consistency reinforces your body's internal clock, promoting better sleep quality over time.

2. Create a Relaxing Bedtime Routine:

Develop a calming pre-sleep routine to signal to your body that it's time to wind down. Activities such as reading, gentle stretching, or practicing relaxation techniques can help transition from the busyness of the day to a more tranquil state.

3. Optimize Sleep Environment:

Ensure your sleep environment is conducive to rest. This includes a comfortable mattress and pillows, as well as a cool, dark, and quiet room. Consider blackout curtains, earplugs, or white noise machines to minimize disruptions.

4. Limit Exposure to Screens Before Bed:

Reduce exposure to blue light from screens at least an hour before bedtime. The light emitted by phones, tablets, and computers can interfere with the production of melatonin, a hormone crucial for sleep.

5. Mindful Nutrition and Hydration:

Be mindful of what and when you eat and drink. Avoid heavy meals, caffeine, and excessive fluids close to bedtime. Opt for a light, balanced snack if you're hungry before sleep.

6. Incorporate Physical Activity:

Regular physical activity can promote better sleep, but it's essential to time it appropriately. Aim for exercise earlier in the day, as intense workouts close to bedtime may have the opposite effect.

7. Manage Stress and Anxiety:

Practice stress-reducing techniques such as meditation, deep breathing, or progressive muscle relaxation.

Managing stress is crucial for mental well-being and can significantly impact the quality of your sleep.

8. Limit Naps:

While short naps can be beneficial, limit them to about 20-30 minutes and avoid napping late in the day to prevent interference with nighttime sleep.

9. Moderate Evening Fluid Intake:

To minimize disruptions during the night, consider reducing your fluid intake in the evening. This can help prevent waking up for bathroom trips and support uninterrupted sleep.

10. Seek Professional Guidance if Needed:

If sleep difficulties persist, consider consulting with a healthcare professional or a sleep specialist. Chronic sleep issues may require a more in-depth evaluation and personalized intervention.

In the intricate dance of physical and mental recovery, optimizing sleep is not a luxury but a necessity. By embracing these principles, you embark on a journey of self-care that nourishes both body and mind, fostering resilience and unlocking the full spectrum of your potential in the waking hours of each new day.

8.2 The impact of sleep on overall well-being:

Sleep is a fundamental pillar of overall well-being, exerting a profound and far-reaching impact on various aspects of physical, mental, and emotional health. The quality and quantity of sleep play a crucial role in maintaining optimal functioning and resilience across diverse dimensions of well-being. Here's a comprehensive exploration of how sleep influences overall health:

1. Physical Restoration and Recovery:
*Cellular Repair: During deep sleep, the body undergoes essential processes of repair and regeneration. Cells are repaired, and growth hormones are released, contributing to overall physical rejuvenation.

*Muscle Recovery: Adequate sleep is vital for the recovery of muscles and tissues, especially after physical activity or exercise. It helps in restoring energy levels and optimizing performance.

2. Cognitive Functioning:

*Memory Consolidation: Sleep is integral to memory consolidation and learning. It enhances the brain's ability to organize and store information acquired during waking hours.

*Problem-Solving and Creativity: Quality sleep is linked to improved cognitive functions, including problem-solving skills, creativity, and the ability to make sound decisions.

3. Emotional Well-Being:

*Mood Regulation: Sleep plays a pivotal role in regulating mood and emotional well-being. Chronic sleep deprivation is associated with an increased risk of mood disorders such as depression and anxiety.

*Stress Resilience: A well-rested mind is more resilient to stress. Sleep deprivation can amplify stress responses, making it harder to cope with daily challenges.

4. Immune Function:

*Immune System Support: Adequate sleep is crucial for a robust immune system. During sleep, the body produces cytokines, proteins that help combat infection and inflammation.

*Illness Prevention: Chronic sleep deprivation has been linked to an increased susceptibility to illnesses, as the immune system may be compromised.

5. Metabolic Health:

*Weight Regulation: Sleep influences appetite-regulating hormones. Lack of sleep may disrupt the balance of hormones that control hunger and satiety, contributing to weight gain.

*Blood Sugar Control: Quality sleep is associated with better blood sugar control, reducing the risk of metabolic disorders such as diabetes.

6. Cardiovascular Health:

*Blood Pressure Regulation: Chronic sleep deprivation has been linked to hypertension and an increased risk of cardiovascular diseases.

*Heart Health: Adequate sleep supports overall cardiovascular health, contributing to a lower risk of heart-related issues.

7. Hormonal Balance:

*Endocrine Function: Sleep influences the secretion of various hormones, including those that regulate stress, growth, and metabolism. Disruptions in sleep patterns can impact hormonal balance.

8. Longevity:

*Life Expectancy: Studies suggest that consistent, high-quality sleep is associated with increased life expectancy. Sleep contributes to overall health and resilience, potentially influencing longevity.

The effect of sleep deprivation on general health can be compared to a symphony, in which every note is resonant throughout the complex network of the mind and body. Ensuring that sleep is prioritized and nurtured is not only a luxury but a crucial part of a holistic approach to health, bringing restoration and vitality from the realm of rest into every waking moment.

CHAPTER 9: BIOHACKING FOR PEAK PERFORMANCE

The pursuit of peak performance has been a timeless undertaking in the broad fabric of human existence, a desire to unleash the entire spectrum of our potential. A phenomenon known as "Biohacking" arises as the avant-garde art of self-mastery in the modern era, when innovation combines with old knowledge. Within this framework, Renaissance Fitness serves as a light, guiding individuals toward the attainment of their full potential.

At its essence, biohacking for peak performance is an intricate dance between science and personal empowerment, a dynamic interplay that transcends conventional boundaries. Renaissance Fitness, as a philosophy, encapsulates the spirit of this movement, embracing the notion that we are not bound by the limitations of our biology but rather empowered to mold and shape it to achieve unparalleled feats.

In the intricate ballet of biohacking, the body becomes a canvas, and technology, nutrition, and mindfulness are the brushes that paint the masterpiece of optimal human performance. The Renaissance Fitness approach recognizes that the mind and body are harmonious partners in this symphony, and to attain peak performance, one must cultivate a holistic balance between mental resilience, physical prowess, and emotional well-being.

Starting on this transforming path requires a dedication to learning about the complexities of one's particular biological composition. It is a desire to grasp the subtleties of our neurological connections and harness the power of nourishment to feed our bodies as temples of energy. Renaissance Fitness enables people to explore the enormous universe of biohacking technologies, which range from wearable gadgets that monitor physiological parameters to advanced dietary regimens suited to specific metabolic demands.

Despite the modern marvels, Renaissance Fitness is a celebration of the ageless knowledge that has echoed down the ages. It is inspired by the Renaissance era, which was characterized by an ardent quest for knowledge and a conviction in humanity's limitless potential. Just as the great minds of the time aspired to transcend restrictions and embrace the whole range of human creativity, Renaissance Fitness encourages individuals to push beyond imagined bounds and strive for the stars of their own potential.

In the modern age, where the demands of life can be relentless and the pace of progress unforgiving, Renaissance Fitness emerges as a sanctuary—a haven where individuals can recalibrate, rejuvenate, and ultimately, rediscover the dormant reservoirs of their inner strength. It is an ode to the human spirit, an affirmation that within each of us lies the capacity for greatness, waiting to be unearthed through the alchemy of biohacking.

As we navigate the uncharted waters of the 21st century, Renaissance Fitness serves as a compass, guiding us toward a future where peak performance is not just an aspiration but a tangible reality. It is an invitation to embrace the journey of self-discovery, to revel in the marvels of modern biohacking, and to unleash the latent potential that resides within each and every one of us in this grand renaissance of human existence.

9.1 Nootropics, supplements, and biohacking techniques:

The world of nootropics, supplements, and biohacking techniques opens the door to improving cognitive function, physical performance, and overall well-being. These technologies serve as beacons of innovation in the search of unlocking the full potential of the human body and mind, giving a plethora of techniques to elevate one's existence.

Nootropics:

Nootropics, often referred to as "smart drugs" or cognitive enhancers, are substances designed to augment cognitive functions such as memory, focus, creativity, and motivation. These compounds work by modulating neurotransmitter levels, enhancing cerebral blood flow, and promoting neuroplasticity. Popular nootropics include:

1. L-Theanine: Found in tea leaves, it promotes relaxation without sedation and complements the stimulating effects of caffeine.

2. Modafinil: Known for its wakefulness-promoting properties, it enhances alertness and cognitive function, often used to combat fatigue.

3. Racetams (e.g., Piracetam): These are a class of nootropics that may enhance memory and learning abilities.

4. Omega-3 Fatty Acids: Essential for brain health, these fatty acids found in fish oil support cognitive function and mood.

5. Adaptogens (e.g., Rhodiola Rosea): These herbs help the body adapt to stress and may improve mental performance.

Supplements:

Supplements are important for covering nutritional gaps, maintaining physical health, and enhancing different biological processes. They may be modified to meet the requirements and aspirations of each individual. The following are important supplements:

1. Vitamin D: Essential for bone health, immune function, and mood regulation. Many people have

insufficient levels, especially in regions with limited sunlight.

2. Magnesium: Supports muscle function, energy production, and relaxation. It is involved in over 300 enzymatic reactions in the body.

3. Protein Powders: Crucial for muscle repair and growth, protein supplements are valuable for individuals engaging in physical activities.

4. Multivitamins: Provide a comprehensive array of essential vitamins and minerals to support overall health and well-being.

5. Collagen: Supports joint, skin, and gut health, promoting overall vitality.

Biohacking Techniques:

Biohacking involves the conscious modification of one's biology through lifestyle changes, environmental adjustments, and the incorporation of cutting-edge technologies. These techniques aim to optimize physical and mental performance:

1. Intermittent Fasting: Cycling between periods of eating and fasting may enhance metabolism, promote autophagy, and improve cognitive function.

2. Sleep Optimization: Prioritizing quality sleep is a foundational biohacking. Adequate rest is crucial for cognitive function, immune health, and overall well-being.

3. Cold Exposure: Cold showers or immersion in cold water can improve circulation, boost the immune system, and increase energy expenditure.

4. Meditation and Mindfulness: Practices such as meditation contribute to stress reduction, improved focus, and emotional well-being.

5. Wearable Technology: Devices like fitness trackers and smartwatches offer real-time data on physical activity, sleep patterns, and other health metrics, empowering individuals to make informed lifestyle choices.

Individuals can carve their own paths to optimal performance and well-being by utilizing the complicated tapestry of nootropics, supplements, and biohacking approaches. This journey is a fluid interplay of science, self-discovery, and a dedication to improving the delicate balance of mind, body, and soul.

9.2 Responsible and ethical biohacking practices:

Responsible and ethical biohacking practices are essential to ensure the well-being of individuals and to uphold ethical standards in the pursuit of optimizing human performance. The field of biohacking, which encompasses a wide range of practices from nootropics to lifestyle interventions, should be approached with a commitment to safety, informed decision-making, and respect for ethical considerations. Here are key principles for responsible and ethical biohacking:

1. Informed Consent:

*People should be aware of the possible dangers, advantages, and uncertainties connected with any biohacking practice.

*Informed consent guarantees that individuals are informed of the possible repercussions of biohacking treatments and are willing to participate in them.

2. Scientific Validity:

*Biohacking practices should be grounded in scientific evidence. Prioritize interventions and supplements with proven efficacy and safety profiles.

*Avoid adopting interventions solely based on anecdotal evidence or unsupported claims.

3. Professional Guidance:

*Seek advice from qualified healthcare professionals, such as doctors, nutritionists, or registered dietitians, before implementing significant biohacking practices.
*Professionals can help assess individual health needs, and potential interactions with existing medications, and provide personalized guidance.

4. Respect for Individual Autonomy:

*Biohacking is a personal journey, and individuals should have the autonomy to choose interventions that align with their values and goals.
*Avoid imposing biohacking practices on others without their informed consent and understanding.

5. Safety First:

*Prioritize safety in all biohacking endeavors. This includes adherence to recommended dosages, awareness of potential side effects, and avoiding practices that pose unnecessary risks.
*Regular monitoring of health metrics and seeking professional guidance can contribute to ensuring safety.

6. Long-Term Health Focus:

*Biohacking practices should be approached with a focus on long-term health and well-being rather than short-term gains.

*Avoid quick-fix approaches that may compromise overall health in the pursuit of immediate results.

7. Open and Transparent Communication:

*Foster open and transparent communication within the biohacking community. Share experiences, both positive and negative, to contribute to collective learning.

*Be cautious about promoting unverified information and emphasize the importance of evidence-based practices.

8. Environmental Sustainability:

*Consider the environmental impact of biohacking practices, such as the production and disposal of supplements and devices.

*Choose sustainable and eco-friendly options when available.

9. Cultural Sensitivity:

*Be mindful of cultural contexts and respect diverse perspectives on health and well-being.

*Avoid promoting biohacking practices that may conflict with cultural or ethical norms.

10. Legal Compliance:

*Adhere to local and international laws and regulations regarding the use of supplements, nootropics, and other biohacking tools.

*Stay informed about any legal restrictions or changes that may impact biohacking practices.

In short, ethical and responsible biohacking is taking a balanced and educated approach that promotes individual well-being, safety, and adherence to ethical norms. Individuals may traverse the biohacking environment with a feeling of responsibility and respect for the field's wider ethical issues by adhering to these guidelines.

CHAPTER 10: CREATING YOUR RENAISSANCE FITNESS LIFESTYLE

There is a great need for self-discovery and self-mastery in the fabric of life, where each thread crafts a unique tale. The pursuit of a Renaissance Fitness Lifestyle emerges as a lighthouse directing individuals towards a harmonious integration of mind, body, and spirit in the present day, distinguished by the unrelenting speed of progress and the unceasing hum of technological breakthroughs.

The concept of Renaissance Fitness transcends the mere physicality of exercise, delving into the realms of holistic well-being and personal transformation. It is an artful tapestry that interlaces the principles of physical fitness, mental resilience, and spiritual nourishment, inviting individuals to step onto the canvas of their own lives and paint a masterpiece of vitality.

At its heart, Renaissance Fitness is an invitation to awaken latent potential inside, much like an undiscovered masterpiece waiting to be uncovered. It is a recognition that our bodies are temples that deserve not only sculpted strength but also careful nurture. In a culture that frequently praises the superficial, Renaissance Fitness promotes a shift in focus – from outward validation to internal fulfillment, from pursuing transient fads to establishing long-term habits.

The journey towards a Renaissance Fitness Lifestyle is a symphony of intentional choices, where each note played is a step towards self-empowerment. It begins with a commitment to physical excellence, where the body becomes a willing canvas for the artistry of discipline and dedication. Strength is not just measured in pounds lifted but in the resilience to persevere, the courage to push boundaries, and the wisdom to honor the body's innate rhythms.

Yet, the Renaissance Fitness Lifestyle is not confined to the walls of a gym; it extends its embrace to the corridors of the mind. Mental fortitude is as crucial as physical prowess, and the pursuit of balance encompasses not only the external but also the internal. Cultivating a Renaissance mindset involves nourishing the intellect, fostering emotional intelligence, and embracing the transformative power of positive affirmations.

In the kaleidoscope of Renaissance Fitness, the spiritual dimension unfurls like a lotus blossom, reaching towards the sunlit realms of self-discovery. It is an acknowledgment that true vitality emanates from a harmonious connection with the inner self, fostering a sense of purpose and aligning one's actions with core values. The practice of mindfulness becomes a compass, guiding individuals through the labyrinth of modernity and grounding them in the present moment.

The Renaissance Fitness Lifestyle is an ode to versatility, an acknowledgment that life's canvas is dynamic, and ever-evolving. It invites individuals to explore diverse modalities of physical activity, be it yoga, strength training, or the meditative dance of martial arts. Just as the Renaissance was a period of rebirth and renewal, this fitness philosophy encourages adaptability, urging individuals to evolve alongside the changing landscapes of their own lives.

In the grand tapestry of existence, the call to embrace a Renaissance Fitness Lifestyle resonates as an anthem of self-empowerment and holistic well-being. It beckons individuals to embark on a journey of self-discovery, where each step is a brushstroke, and each choice is a stroke of the artist's hand. As the Renaissance unfolded through the ages, so too can the canvas of our lives unfurl, revealing the masterpiece that lies within — a testament to the boundless potential that awaits those who dare to embark on this transformative journey.

10.1 Developing a personalized fitness and wellness routine:

Creating a personalized fitness and wellness routine is a rewarding journey that considers individual goals, preferences, and overall well-being. Here's a step-by-step guide to help you develop a routine tailored to your unique needs:

1. Define Your Goals:

Identify specific, measurable, achievable, relevant, and time-bound (SMART) goals. Whether it's weight loss, muscle gain, increased flexibility, or stress reduction, clarity in your objectives will guide your routine.

2. Assess Your Current Fitness Level:

Understand your starting point by assessing your fitness level. Consider factors like endurance, strength, flexibility, and balance. This self-awareness will help you choose appropriate exercises and track progress effectively.

3. Choose Activities You Enjoy:

Opt for exercises that resonate with your interests. Whether it's swimming, dancing, hiking, or weightlifting, enjoying your workouts increases adherence and makes the journey more fulfilling.

4. Create a Balanced Routine:

Include a mix of cardiovascular exercises, strength training, flexibility work, and relaxation techniques. This balance ensures comprehensive fitness and minimizes the risk of overtraining or neglecting certain aspects.

5. Set a Realistic Schedule:

Determine how much time you can realistically commit to your routine each week. Consistency is key, so choose a schedule that aligns with your daily life and allows for sustainable progress.

6. Start Gradually:

If you're new to exercising or returning after a break, begin with manageable intensity and duration. Gradually increase the challenge to avoid burnout or injury.

7. Incorporate Strength Training:

Include strength training exercises to improve muscle tone, boost metabolism, and enhance overall functional fitness. Focus on major muscle groups and gradually progress in resistance.

8. Prioritize Cardiovascular Health:

Integrate cardiovascular exercises like jogging, cycling, or dancing to enhance heart health, stamina, and calorie burn. Aim for at least 150 minutes of moderate-intensity cardio per week.

9. Include Flexibility and Mobility Work:

Dedicate time to stretch and improve flexibility. Activities like yoga or Pilates enhance mobility, reduce the risk of injuries, and contribute to a well-rounded routine.

10. Mind-Body Connection:

Incorporate mindfulness practices such as meditation or deep breathing exercises. These techniques can help manage stress, improve focus, and enhance overall mental well-being.

11. Hydration and Nutrition:

Support your fitness routine with a balanced diet and proper hydration. Consult with a nutritionist to align your dietary choices with your fitness goals.

12. Rest and Recovery:

Allow time for rest and recovery. Adequate sleep, rest days, and activities like foam rolling contribute to muscle recovery and overall well-being.

13. Monitor and Adjust:

Regularly assess your progress and be willing to adjust your routine. Adapt to changes in your goals, preferences, and lifestyle to maintain motivation and enjoyment.

14. Seek Professional Guidance:

Consider consulting with fitness professionals, such as personal trainers or health experts, to create a customized plan and ensure proper form and technique.

Keep in mind that every person's fitness journey is different. The secret is to discover a routine that suits your specific needs and makes the journey to wellness enjoyable and long-lasting.

10.2 Sustaining long-term health and vitality:

Long-term health and vitality need a delicate dance of lifestyle choices, mindful practices, and a sincere dedication to supporting the body, mind, and spirit. In a society where the demands of everyday existence may easily eclipse the value of overall well-being, the quest for enduring health becomes an art – a continuous masterpiece crafted with purposeful decisions and mindful living.

At the heart of sustaining long-term health and vitality lies the recognition that the body is a temple deserving of mindful care. This involves adopting a balanced and nutritious diet that serves as the foundation for physical well-being. Choosing whole, unprocessed foods provides the body with the essential nutrients it craves, fostering resilience and fortifying against the challenges of time.

Physical activity emerges as a stalwart companion on the journey to sustained health. It is not merely a means to an end but a celebration of the body's capabilities, a symphony of movement that extends beyond the confines of structured exercise. Engaging in activities that bring joy — whether it be a leisurely stroll, invigorating dance, or the tranquility of yoga — transforms exercise from a task into a delightful ritual, ensuring its integration into the tapestry of everyday life.

Equally pivotal in the mosaic of sustained health is the cultivation of mental resilience. In a world rife with stressors, nurturing mental well-being becomes a cornerstone for vitality. Practices such as mindfulness meditation, deep-breathing exercises, and the cultivation of positive thought patterns create a sanctuary for the mind, fostering emotional equilibrium and shielding against the wear and tear of daily challenges.

However, the importance of long-term health and vitality extends beyond the physical and mental dimensions, all the way to the spiritual center. This may not always imply adhering to a certain religious theory, but rather a discovery of one's inner self, a connection to a feeling of purpose that burns the soul. Engaging in fulfilling activities, cultivating meaningful friendships, and experiencing moments of thankfulness all contribute to a profound feeling of holistic wholeness.

The path to long-term health and vitality is fraught with ups and downs, emphasizing the significance of adaptation. Life is a living fabric, and as the seasons change, so must our attitude to happiness. Listening to the body's messages, being aware of its changing demands, and making intentional modifications to lifestyle choices as circumstances change are all part of it.

Maintaining long-term health and vitality becomes a monument to self-love and self-respect as the brushstrokes of time paint the canvas of our lives. It's an acknowledgment that the journey is just as essential as the goal and that each day is a new chance to perfect the masterpiece that is our well-being. Individuals may build a road towards prolonged health and vitality via purposeful decisions, nourishing practices, and a firm dedication to the art of living — a journey that unfolds as a timeless hymn to the lasting power and tenacity of the human spirit.

CONCLUSION

As we reach the final pages of Renaissance Fitness: Unleashing Your Potential in the Modern Age, The path to optimal well-being is evidently a complicated tapestry woven with threads of physical strength, mental resilience, and a thorough awareness of our bodies in the context of the modern world. We have gone into the worlds of ancient wisdom, cutting-edge research, and practical tactics to empower individuals on their quest for holistic health in our Renaissance Fitness investigation.

The Renaissance era was characterized by a revival of art, culture, and intellectual curiosity, and in many ways, we find ourselves standing at the threshold of a similar rebirth in the domain of fitness. Our understanding of the human body has evolved, blending age-old principles with contemporary research, and the result is a comprehensive approach that transcends mere physical appearance. Fitness, in this modern age, is not just about sculpting our bodies; it is about nurturing our minds, fostering resilience, and embracing a holistic lifestyle.

Throughout this book, we have explored the importance of a balanced approach to fitness—one that encompasses physical exercise, mindful nutrition, and the cultivation of mental well-being. The Renaissance Fitness paradigm encourages us to move beyond the limitations of fad diets and extreme workout regimens, emphasizing sustainability and long-term vitality. It is a call to action, urging individuals to become architects of their own well-being, understanding that the path to optimal health is as unique as each individual.

As we say goodbye to these pages, let us carry the spirit of Renaissance Fitness with us—a dedication to self-discovery, an understanding of the interdependence of mind and body, and a readiness to adapt to the ever-changing landscape of wellness. In today's world, when the demands of everyday life can be overwhelming, adopting a Renaissance approach to fitness becomes a beacon of light, directing us towards balance, strength, and fulfillment.

May this book serve as a catalyst for change—a roadmap to unlock the vast potential that resides within each one of us. As we embark on our individual journeys, let us remember that the pursuit of Renaissance Fitness is not a destination but a continuous evolution—a dynamic process of growth and self-discovery that transcends the boundaries of time.

In the spirit of the Renaissance, let us celebrate the diversity of our bodies, minds, and experiences, and may our collective commitment to holistic well-being usher in an era where fitness is not merely a goal but a way of life—a journey of self-empowerment that knows no bounds.